Copyright © 2019 by John Wood MD

All rights reserved. No part of this publication may be reproduced, distributed, or transmitted in any form or by any means, including photocopying, recording, or other electronic or mechanical methods, without the prior written permission of the publisher, except in the case of brief quotations embodied in critical reviews and certain other noncommercial uses permitted by copyright law

Table of Contents

Introduction 4

What is cbd oil 6

   Why did humans start using cannabis 6

   How are hemp and marijuana different 7

   What's the difference between THC and CBD 8

   What are terpenes, and why are they important 10

   What are the benefits of taking CBD 10

   What's the difference between hemp oil and hemp oil with CBD 15

   CBD extraction method 16

   What's the best way to take hemp oil with CBD 18

   What's the correct dose of CBD 19

   What's the difference between CBD isolate and full-spectrum CBD oil 20

   What are the potential side effects of CBD oil 22

   How do you know you're getting your money's worth 23

   Will I get high from using CBD 25

   Will using CBD make me fail a drug test 26

What is diabetes 29

   Diabetes types 29

   Symptoms of diabetes 30

   Causes of diabetes 32

- Diabetes risk factors 34
- Diabetes complications 35
- Treatment of diabetes 37
- Diabetes and diet 39
- Diabetes diagnosis 41
- Diabetes prevention 43
- Diabetes in pregnancy 44
- Diabetes in children 45

Cbd oil for diabetes 46
- CBD Impact on Diabetes 47
- Clinical Studies 50
- Clinical Trials in the Pipeline 52
- CBD Oil Dosage for Diabetes 53
- CBD Dosage for Mild Diabetes Symptoms 54
- Best cbd oil for diabetes 56

Final Thoughts on Finding the Best CBD Oil for Diabetes 64

Introduction

You probably don't have to look farther than your local drugstore or beauty product supplier to know CBD has taken a starring role in everything from sparkling water and gummies to tincture oils and lotions. Some may even say that CBD is the "it" ingredient of this day and age.

You've probably also heard that CBD which is an abbreviation for cannabidiol can help with stress, anxiety, and pain. "When people are in pain, they have a stress response, which causes an increase in cortisol and an increase in blood sugar," says Veronica J. Brady, PhD, CDE, a registered nurse and an assistant professor at the Cizik School of Nursing at the University of Texas in Houston. Relieving pain can help alleviate the stress response and improve blood sugar levels, as well as improve sleep, she adds.

If you're managing type 2 diabetes, it's natural to be curious about whether CBD might help you manage those symptoms, too, to help stabilize your blood sugar. Some healthcare professionals say CBD may play a role in treating diabetes, but it's important to understand that the only health condition CBD has proved effective for is epilepsy in kids. The jury is unfortunately still out, because of a lack of comprehensive research on CBD and type 2 diabetes.

"We don't know that THC or CBD exerts an effect on diabetes itself, and that means control of blood sugars," says Cory Toth, MD, a neurologist at Fraser Health at Burnaby Hospital in British Columbia. He adds that pain relief is the number one reason people with diabetes use CBD and tetrahydrocannabinol (THC), another compound found in cannabis, in Canada. It's worth noting that CBD does not cause psychoactive effects like THC, its chemical cousin.

What is cbd oil

Why did humans start using cannabis

Cannabis sativa was one of the earliest plants cultivated by humankind. The very first use of cannabis was documented in China around 4000 BC. A very versatile plant, it was used for food, medicine, religious and spiritual rituals, industrial fiber, and, of course, recreation.

From China, cannabis spread to India, the Arabian Peninsula, and then on to Europe with the spice trade. Through European colonization, use of cannabis spread to the Americas, Caribbean, and throughout the world. How the plant was used depended on the variety of cannabis, the parts of the plant, and how the plant was cultivated.

The variety of cannabis known as hemp was traditionally valued primarily for its fibers with high tensile strength, making it ideal for creating rope and textiles. Hemp seeds and sprouts were eaten as a good source of high-quality protein and beneficial omega-3 fatty acids. The variety of cannabis known as marijuana was specifically cultivated for the euphoric properties of THC, which is concentrated mostly in the flower buds of the plant. Only recently have the unique medicinal properties of both hemp and marijuana been fully recognized.

How are hemp and marijuana different

Cannabis sativa has several alter egos, but marijuana and hemp are the two best known. Though both plants look the same, their chemical composition is quite different.

The chemical difference has to do with the presence or absence of certain enzymes. Both marijuana and hemp contain a chemical substance called cannabigerol (CBGA), which is concentrated mostly in the flower buds of the plant. Marijuana contains an enzyme that converts CBGA into THC; hemp contains a different enzyme that converts CBGA into CBD (cannabidiol).

Whereas marijuana contains both THC and CBD, hemp contains almost exclusively CBD THC occurs only in very trace amounts. Remember, though, that there are many varieties of marijuana and hemp plants, and their concentrations of THC and CBD vary. Those with high THC are used primarily for recreational use; plants with low or no THC and high CBD are best for medicinal use. Only cannabis with less than 0.3% THC can be legally classified as hemp.

What's the difference between THC and CBD

Both THC (in marijuana) and CBD (in hemp) belong to a class of plant chemical compounds called cannabinoids. There are different receptors for cannabinoid compounds located throughout the body.

For instance, CB1 receptors are found in high concentrations in the brain and nervous system. CB2 receptors are located throughout the body, but predominantly within the lower body and immune system.

THC's intoxicating powers come from its ability to mimic anandamide, an endocannabinoid or naturally occurring mood-altering substance in the body that binds to CB1 receptors in the brain and is associated with having a rosy disposition. THC binds to anandamide's CB1 receptors even more tightly than anandamide itself, triggering an exaggerated or euphoric response — in other words, you get high.

Compared to THC, CBD has very different properties. It weakly binds to both CB1 and CB2 receptors in the brain and body, gently stimulating and blocking them at the same time. This not only mildly activates the receptors, but is also thought to trigger the body to create more CB1 and CB2 receptors, a process known as upregulation. It also results in increased natural levels of anandamide.

When the body experiences an increase in CB receptors, it becomes more sensitive to the natural endocannabinoids (anandamide and others) already present in the body. The end result of taking CBD is an uplifted mood and improved pain tolerance without an exaggerated euphoric response, so you don't get high when you use it.

CBD also modulates other receptors in the body. For instance, modulation of the 5-HT1A receptor (involved with serotonin, a mood hormone) provides mood-balancing properties: It's calming, but not highly sedating, so it's considered neutral — though it often results in improved sleep for many people. Another example is modulation of opioid receptors, which provides pain relief and tissue-supporting properties.

Beyond THC and CBD, Cannabis sativa plants contain over a hundred other cannabinoids that have a similar effect as CBD, but milder THC is the only one known to be intoxicating. Cannabis plants also possess a wide spectrum of different chemical components offering a range of medicinal properties.

What are terpenes, and why are they important

Aside from cannabinoids, one of the most prominent chemicals in cannabis plants is terpenes, organic and aromatic compounds found in essential oils. Interestingly, it's the terpenes that give marijuana its distinct "weedy" odor and taste, not the cannabinoids.

Terpenes are beneficial on their own. For instance, research in the British Journal of Pharmacology found that terpenes are gastro-protective, suggesting they may be beneficial to people with ulcers, and that they have anti-inflammatory properties.

Also important is terpenes' ability to enhance the properties of CBD. This phenomenon, called the "entourage effect," is considered by many experts in the industry to be essential for gaining the full benefit of the plant. It also points to the importance of using a full-spectrum extract of hemp, which provides a full range of chemical components including terpenes, as opposed to purified CBD or CBD isolate, which contains only CBD.

What are the benefits of taking CBD

Cannabinoids, including cannabidiol (CBD), work by mimicking natural endocannabinoids like anandamide (described above) in the body. Endocannabinoids are part of a complex messaging system in the body called the endocannabinoid system. The endocannabinoid system oversees or regulates parts of the nervous system, endorphins, immune system functions, hormones, mood and emotions, metabolism, and many other chemical messengers in the body.

My mimicking endocannabinoids, CBD offers a wide range of benefits, including:

- Decreased pain
- Enhanced sense of well-being
- Increased calm
- Improved sleep
- Reduced stress (thanks to CBD's adaptogenic properties, which make you more resistant to various types of stress)

But because CBD doesn't cause euphoria or impair motor skills, you can use it any time of the day or evening. Let's explore in more detail how it works for various health concerns.

Nervous system conditions

Like other cannabinoids, CBD readily crosses the blood brain barrier, making it ideal for affecting central nervous system conditions. CBD helps calm the nervous system, reduces inflammation, and is strongly neuroprotective. Not surprisingly, clinical studies evaluating cannabidiol for treatment of anxiety, post traumatic stress disorder (PTSD), seizure disorders (especially childhood seizures), and even schizophrenia have shown remarkable effectiveness.

Chronic Pain

Management of chronic pain is another application for which CBD is ideally suited, and it works in a number of ways. It and other non-THC cannabinoids found in hemp flower-bud extracts work to block pain-conducting nerve impulses, which reduces your perception of pain. Stimulation of CB1 in the brain increases dopamine, which counteracts pain. Just as importantly, these same chemical substances reduce inflammation, the driving force behind pain, which allows healing to occur. CBD and other cannabinoids also reduce pain by affecting endorphins, the feel-good chemicals we naturally produce to suppress pain. Unlike opioids (heroin, narcotics), which mimic endorphins and ultimately suppress natural endorphins, cannabinoids modulate endorphins.

This means, in effect, that CBD and cannabinoids increase natural endorphins. So instead of causing dependence and addiction like opioids, CBD and cannabinoids do the opposite — so much so that CBD has proven valuable for countering narcotic and cocaine addiction. From a medicinal standpoint, the fact that CBD has the potential to relieve pain without causing euphoria, intoxication, or addiction makes it an intriguing therapeutic option — it has high potential for being at least a partial solution to the current opioid epidemic.

Immune dysfunction + chronic illness

CBD and other chemical substances in hemp flower-bud extracts are strong immune system modulators. This means they control inflammation throughout the body, and also fine-tune the immune system for optimal performance. This combined with CBD's ability to ease pain and anxiety make it an ideal consideration for illnesses associated with immune dysfunction, including fibromyalgia, chronic fatigue syndrome, chronic Lyme disease, and autoimmune illnesses.

Gut dysfunction

The immunomodulation benefits of CBD and cannabinoids extend to the GI tract. CBD may have value in treating inflammatory bowel diseases, including Crohn's disease and ulcerative colitis, but that value is still being defined by clinical studies.

Cancer symptoms

The wide range of benefits associated with cannabis have garnered interest for use in cancer therapy. Research suggests that cannabinoids, including CBD, may have anti-tumor effects. While this is not enough to define cannabis as a treatment for cancer, it does make it attractive as a complement to other therapies, for both reducing symptoms and possibly enhancing the effects of anticancer drugs.

Additional health concerns

The benefits of CBD and other non-THC cannabinoids don't stop there. Terpenes and the wide spectrum of other chemical compounds found in hemp flower-bud extracts provide potent anti-inflammatory and antioxidant properties. And like most other herbs, hemp flower-bud extracts have been associated with antimicrobial properties, though cannabis doesn't appear to be as strong an antimicrobial as many other herbs.

What's the difference between hemp oil and hemp oil with CBD

This is a common source of confusion. Many people see hemp oil on grocery store shelves and assume or wonder if it contains CBD and other cannabinoids. Adding to the confusion, CBD products are often sold as hemp oil, and CBD oil is often mixed with hemp oil.

But make no mistake, hemp oil and hemp oil with CBD (or CBD oil) are not the same. The hemp oil you might see on grocery store shelves is made by cold pressing hemp seeds. It's high in omega-3 fatty acids and other beneficial fatty acids, but hemp oil found in the grocery store does not contain significant amounts of cannabinoids including THC or CBD. While hemp oil is a healthful option for a salad dressing, it has no medicinal value by itself.

Cannabinoids, including CBD in hemp and THC in marijuana, are most highly concentrated in the flower buds, not the seeds. These chemical components of the plant must be extracted from the flower buds to be useful.

CBD extraction method

For medicinal use, cannabinoids are extracted from hemp and concentrated into a thick oil that, when ingested, elevates blood levels of cannabinoids for a more sustained period of time. (That's compared to inhaling vaporized marijuana, where THC dissipates from blood quickly, making it ideal for recreational use.) CBD oil from hemp contains CBD and other cannabinoids, along with terpenes and other chemical components. It contains only trace amounts of THC (<0.3%).

The four main methods of CBD extraction

Alcohol extraction: The most common method, chemical extraction uses alcohol or hexane as solvents. The solvent is dried off, leaving the dense oil — and possibly harmful residual solvents — behind.

Hydrocarbon extraction: This method primarily uses propane, butane, or a mix of the two as solvents. A very effective method for extracting the full spectrum of cannabinoids and terpenes in hemp, it delivers a highly potent product. However, because propane is extremely flammable, hydrocarbon extraction requires a high degree of expertise and safety; a lack of expertise could result in solvent residues in the final CBD product. For that reason, if you choose a CBD product made with this method, just be sure the company also provides a test report or Certificate of Analysis (COA) showing the product is safe to consume.

CO2 extraction: A newer method, CO2 extraction is done without using chemical solvents. Instead, it uses carbon dioxide to extract the full range of chemical components from the flower buds and then distill them into dense CBD oil.

Thermal Extraction: This method uses hot air to safely vaporize the full spectrum of chemical components at high concentration from the buds, and then the vapor is distilled into CBD oil. This method also activates the cannabinoids by removing an extra carboxyl ring from their molecular chain (a chemical reaction called decarboxylation), enabling them to interact directly with CB receptors for maximal medicinal value. And it preserves the native terpenes, which are beneficial on their own, and also enhance the properties of CBD via the entourage effect.

Lipid-based extraction: This method uses fats such as organic coconut oil to absorb and encapsulate the plant's chemical compounds. The upsides of lipid-based extraction are that the fat helps make the CBD more bioavailable (easy to absorb), and there are no harsh solvents used. The downside: you won't get a full spectrum of compounds like you would with vapor distillation or CO2 extraction.

What's the best way to take hemp oil with CBD

Condensed CBD oil can be taken as a thick paste, but this is the least pleasant option. More commonly, the CBD oil is mixed with a carrier oil, such as hemp oil or coconut oil, to a specific concentration of CBD. The distinctive taste — which comes from the terpenes and not the cannabinoids — is often masked with chocolate, mint, or other flavorings. It typically comes in a small bottle with a dropper to administer the oil mixture.

The best way to take CBD oil mixed with a carrier oil to a specific concentration is to place a few drops or dropperfuls under your tongue for 15 seconds to access the sublingual gland. There, the CBD is absorbed directly into the bloodstream (called sublingual consumption or administration) for the fastest acting effects.

Another method is to take a few drops or dropperfuls orally, swish the liquid around in your mouth, and then swallow it. With this method, CBD's chemical components are absorbed through mucous membranes of the mouth and intestinal tract directly into the bloodstream.

CBD oil mixed with a carrier oil can also be taken as soft-gel capsules to avoid any taste, but absorption is only through the intestinal tract. This decreases the oil's potential benefits, because some of the chemical components may be broken down by digestion before being absorbed.

What's the correct dose of CBD

The average dose range is 10-50 mg of CBD, one to three times per day, though much higher doses of 100-200 mg (sometimes required to control pain) are equally well tolerated. Some people will notice benefit at the lower end of the dose range, but most people will need 15-30 mg to notice any effects. Because different products provide different concentrations of CBD, the packaging usually states how much CBD is in the entire bottle as opposed to the amount in a certain number of drops or dropperfuls, so measuring can be a little tricky.

If you're taking the oil in liquid form, one dropperful of a low concentration product (100 mg CBD per fluid ounce) will provide about 3 mg of CBD per dropperful not enough to notice any significant effects. A dropperful of the medium grade product (500 mg of CBD per fluid ounce) will deliver about 15 mg of CBD — a good starting dose. And a dropperful of a high concentration product (1500 mg CBD per fluid ounce) will provide about 50 mg of CBD per dropperful.

How many milligrams of CBD is in your 1 ML dose?

CBD oil is also available as soft gel capsules. With these, the mg quantity of CBD should be designated per capsule. Because some of the chemical compounds in capsules are lost during digestion, you may find you need to take a little more to experience the benefits.

As with any medicinal herb, start at a low dose and gradually build up to a higher dose as you get used to the effects of the substance. Most people notice benefits almost immediately, but some experts suggest that full benefit does not occur until after a couple of weeks of consecutive use.

What's the difference between CBD isolate and full-spectrum CBD oil

A lot. CBD isolate (which is CBD alone) acts very differently in the body than a spectrum of hemp chemical components. Here are some quick definitions: CBD isolate is purified cannabidiol (CBD) without any other chemical components of hemp. Usually purity is a good thing, but in this case, purified CBD is missing all of the other beneficial compounds the hemp plant has to offer.

Full-spectrum CBD oil contains cannabidiol, plus the full spectrum of other components of the whole plant, including trace amounts of THC (at less than 0.3%), other cannabinoids, and terpenes.

Broad-spectrum CBD oil is full-spectrum CBD with the THC removed. It's not as effective as full-spectrum CBD oil with trace THC.

The cannabis plant naturally generates cannabinoids, terpenes, and other chemical compounds to serve different functions in the plant. These functions include regulatory properties, potent antioxidants, and protection from microbes and insects. Any creature that consumes the chemicals from the plant gains these same benefits.

You can think of the full spectrum of all the chemical compounds found in cannabis as the "language" of the plant. It's not one chemical, but all the chemicals combined working together that cause a response (again, the entourage effect). When you consume CBD oil, you gain the benefits of all those chemical substances in natural synergy. For that reason, you get full benefit at a dose range of 25-50 mg.

CBD isolate is limited to that single chemical messenger. The synergy provided by the full spectrum of chemicals in CBD oil is lost. This is likely why clinical studies using purified CBD require very high doses, in the range of 750-1500 mg of CBD several times daily, to see a benefit.

When CBD is formally legalized at the national level, prescription drugs providing high doses of purified CBD will become available (several are already in the pipeline). CBD drugs will likely be very costly, require very high doses of CBD isolate, and will likely not provide the same benefits as full-spectrum CBD oil.

What are the potential side effects of CBD oil

Reported side effects of hemp oil with CBD are generally mild and uncommon and can include tiredness, loose stools, and mild changes in appetite and weight (either increased or decreased). Both hemp oil with CBD (hemp flower-bud extracts) and purified CBD (CBD isolate) have been shown in both animal and human clinical trials to be remarkably safe and well tolerated.

Prolonged use is not associated with an increased risk of side effects. In research studies, up to 1500 mg of purified CBD per day has been used to address various medical illnesses without reported harmful effects including changes in heart rate, blood pressure, temperature, oxygen and carbon dioxide levels, electrolyte balance, gastrointestinal function, psychomotor functions, or sleep cycles.

Prolonged use at high doses has not shown potential for abuse of CBD. In fact, a clinical study published in 2018 found that recreational polydrug users did not show abuse potential with use of CBD. Long-term studies have not evaluated potential changes in hormonal balance or long-term adverse changes in liver function, though prolonged use of CBD enhances metabolism of certain drugs. Stopping CBD oil suddenly has not been associated with withdrawal effects.

How do you know you're getting your money's worth

While the cost of CBD oil products is presently high, it will likely come down dramatically after CBD and hemp are legal by federal standards but prices will still vary widely. A high price for a CBD product does not always imply high quality, though a low price generally indicates you're not getting enough CBD to see a benefit, so it's important to know what to look for when buying or using a product.

Reputable companies selling CBD oil products will state the CBD concentration and extraction methods on the bottle or website. Typically, the concentration is stated as milligrams (mg) of CBD per fluid ounce (though some products standardize mg of CBD to milliliters (ml). The benefit comes from the amount of CBD consumed, not the amount of oil.

To calculate the cost per milligram of CBD, simply divide the dollar amount of the product by the total milligrams of CBD in the bottle. So for instance, a product with 600 mg CBD in a 1 fluid-ounce bottle costing $80 is equal to about 13 cents per mg of CBD; a product with 100 mg of CBD in the same size bottle selling for $40 works out to 40 cents per mg of CBD. In this case, it pays to splurge on the $80 bottle.

As for extraction methods, remember that thermal extraction and CO_2 extraction are preferred. These methods yield a full-spectrum CBD product, which will likely be more costly than a CBD isolate because it's significantly more beneficial. Alcohol extraction is a cheaper method that pulls a more narrow spectrum of plant chemicals and higher levels of chlorophyll, which doesn't taste great and also takes up space where more CBD could be. Lipid-based extractions will likely fall in the middle price-wise.

The highest quality cannabis is grown indoors, so quality standards can be controlled. Use of clean water and organic methods of farming that are free of pesticide use and unnatural fertilizers are, of course, preferred. With outdoor-farmed cannabis, quality standards and potency are not as easily controlled.

Taste can be a sign of value, too. Poor quality oils will have a very unpleasant chemical taste, and they can cause significant burning to mouth tissues. A good quality product should be smooth and not cause significant burning. Interestingly, the best quality products are associated with a distinct cannabis taste, indicating that the full spectrum of chemical components (with trace levels of THC) are present.

Will I get high from using CBD

No. Even in high doses, CBD oil will not cause euphoria or impair coordination, balance, or motor functions. Psychoactive effects start at 3-5% THC; CBD products contain less than 0.3% THC.

Use of CBD oil is associated with improved sense of well-being, but not an exaggerated feeling of well-being. Use of CBD oil has never been associated with hallucinations or abnormal mental activity.

Will using CBD make me fail a drug test

The trace amount of THC in CBD oil (<0.3%) is not enough to trigger most drug tests as being positive for THC. You would need to consume about 1000-2000 mg per day of CBD to fail a drug test for THC if the employer is testing to SAMHSA guidelines (Substance Abuse and Mental Health Services Administration). If you are tested regularly and taking high doses of CBD, and you are concerned about the very low risk of a positive drug test for THC associated with using hemp-derived products, you could opt to use purified CBD, which does not contain anything but CBD. Just know that purified CBD doesn't provide the same spectrum of benefits as CBD oil.

Can you overdose on cannabis?

There have been no reports of anyone overdosing on cannabis. One of the unique properties of the chemical components of cannabis, including both hemp and marijuana, is that they don't cause respiratory or cardiac depression. This sets even recreational use of cannabis widely apart from narcotics and alcohol, both of which can cause severe respiratory depression and death at excessive doses. Excessive doses of hemp, and more especially, marijuana, may make you very agitated and feel terrible, but there are no known deaths from cannabis overdose.

Are foods and beverages with purified CBD safe?

Many food and beverage companies are already taking advantage of the growing CBD trend and adding CBD to food and beverage products, though the practice is not approved by the FDA. They are mostly using purified CBD (CBD isolate) instead of CBD oil, because purified CBD has no significant taste and comes from poorer quality hemp, which is cheaper to produce. Whether it's completely safe is totally unknown. Using CBD in defined doses for medicinal purposes is one thing, but putting it in food and beverages is something entirely different. Someone may wind up getting CBD from multiple products, and so their daily dose could vary significantly. Taking a standardized dose of CBD oil daily as a recognized medicinal is a very different thing from taking uncontrolled doses of CBD isolate daily infused artificially into food and beverage products, and the long term risk may be very different — no one really knows for sure.

What is diabetes

Diabetes types

Diabetes mellitus, commonly known as diabetes, is a metabolic disease that causes high blood sugar. The hormone insulin moves sugar from the blood into your cells to be stored or used for energy. With diabetes, your body either doesn't make enough insulin or can't effectively use the insulin it does make. Untreated high blood sugar from diabetes can damage your nerves, eyes, kidneys, and other organs.

There are a few different types of diabetes:

Type 1 diabetes is an autoimmune disease. The immune system attacks and destroys cells in the pancreas, where insulin is made. It's unclear what causes this attack. About 10 percent of people with diabetes have this type.

Type 2 diabetes occurs when your body becomes resistant to insulin, and sugar builds up in your blood.

Prediabetes occurs when your blood sugar is higher than normal, but it's not high enough for a diagnosis of type 2 diabetes.

Gestational diabetes is high blood sugar during pregnancy. Insulin-blocking hormones produced by the placenta cause this type of diabetes.

A rare condition called diabetes insipidus is not related to diabetes mellitus, although it has a similar name. It's a different condition in which your kidneys remove too much fluid from your body.

Each type of diabetes has unique symptoms, causes, and treatments. Learn more about how these types differ from one another.

Symptoms of diabetes

Diabetes symptoms are caused by rising blood sugar.

General symptoms

The general symptoms of diabetes include:

- increased hunger
- increased thirst
- weight loss
- frequent urination
- blurry vision
- extreme fatigue

- sores that don't heal

Symptoms in men

In addition to the general symptoms of diabetes, men with diabetes may have a decreased sex drive, erectile dysfunction (ED), and poor muscle strength.

Symptoms in women

Women with diabetes can also have symptoms such as urinary tract infections, yeast infections, and dry, itchy skin.

Type 1 diabetes

Symptoms of type 1 diabetes can include:

- extreme hunger
- increased thirst
- unintentional weight loss
- frequent urination
- blurry vision
- tiredness
- It may also result in mood changes.

Type 2 diabetes

Symptoms of type 2 diabetes can include:

- increased hunger
- increased thirst
- increased urination
- blurry vision
- tiredness
- sores that are slow to heal
- It may also cause recurring infections. This is because elevated glucose levels make it harder for the body to heal.

Gestational diabetes

Most women with gestational diabetes don't have any symptoms. The condition is often detected during a routine blood sugar test or oral glucose tolerance test that is usually performed between the 24th and 28th weeks of gestation. In rare cases, a woman with gestational diabetes will also experience increased thirst or urination.

Causes of diabetes

Different causes are associated with each type of diabetes.

Type 1 diabetes

Doctors don't know exactly what causes type 1 diabetes. For some reason, the immune system mistakenly attacks and destroys insulin-producing beta cells in the pancreas. Genes may play a role in some people. It's also possible that a virus sets off the immune system attack.

Type 2 diabetes

Type 2 diabetes stems from a combination of genetics and lifestyle factors. Being overweight or obese increases your risk too. Carrying extra weight, especially in your belly, makes your cells more resistant to the effects of insulin on your blood sugar. This condition runs in families. Family members share genes that make them more likely to get type 2 diabetes and to be overweight.

Gestational diabetes

Gestational diabetes is the result of hormonal changes during pregnancy. The placenta produces hormones that make a pregnant woman's cells less sensitive to the effects of insulin. This can cause high blood sugar during pregnancy.

Women who are overweight when they get pregnant or who gain too much weight during their pregnancy are more likely to get gestational diabetes.

Diabetes risk factors

Certain factors increase your risk for diabetes.

Type 1 diabetes

You're more likely to get type 1 diabetes if you're a child or teenager, you have a parent or sibling with the condition, or you carry certain genes that are linked to the disease.

Type 2 diabetes

Your risk for type 2 diabetes increases if you:

- are overweight
- are age 45 or older
- have a parent or sibling with the condition
- aren't physically active
- have had gestational diabetes
- have prediabetes
- have high blood pressure, high cholesterol, or high triglycerides
- have African American, Hispanic or Latino American, Alaska Native, Pacific Islander, American Indian, or Asian American ancestry

Gestational diabetes

Your risk for gestational diabetes increases if you:

- are overweight
- are over age 25
- had gestational diabetes during a past pregnancy
- have given birth to a baby weighing more than 9 pounds
- have a family history of type 2 diabetes
- have polycystic ovary syndrome (PCOS)

Diabetes complications

High blood sugar damages organs and tissues throughout your body. The higher your blood sugar is and the longer you live with it, the greater your risk for complications. Complications associated with diabetes include:

- heart disease, heart attack, and stroke
- neuropathy
- nephropathy
- retinopathy and vision loss
- hearing loss
- foot damage such as infections and sores that don't heal
- skin conditions such as bacterial and fungal infections
- depression

- dementia

Gestational diabetes

Uncontrolled gestational diabetes can lead to problems that affect both the mother and baby. Complications affecting the baby can include:

- premature birth
- higher-than-normal weight at birth
- increased risk for type 2 diabetes later in life
- low blood sugar
- jaundice
- stillbirth

The mother can develop complications such as high blood pressure (preeclampsia) or type 2 diabetes. She may also require cesarean delivery, commonly referred to as a C-section. The mother's risk of gestational diabetes in future pregnancies also increases.

Treatment of diabetes

Doctors treat diabetes with a few different medications. Some of these drugs are taken by mouth, while others are available as injections.

Type 1 diabetes

Insulin is the main treatment for type 1 diabetes. It replaces the hormone your body isn't able to produce. There are four types of insulin that are most commonly used. They're differentiated by how quickly they start to work, and how long their effects last:

Rapid-acting insulin starts to work within 15 minutes and its effects last for 3 to 4 hours.

Short-acting insulin starts to work within 30 minutes and lasts 6 to 8 hours.

Intermediate-acting insulin starts to work within 1 to 2 hours and lasts 12 to 18 hours.

Long-acting insulin starts to work a few hours after injection and lasts 24 hours or longer.

Type 2 diabetes

Diet and exercise can help some people manage type 2 diabetes. If lifestyle changes aren't enough to lower your blood sugar, you'll need to take medication.

These drugs lower your blood sugar in a variety of ways:

Types of drug	How they work	Example(s)
Alpha-glucosidase inhibitors	Slow your body's breakdown of sugars and starchy foods	Acarbose (Precose) and miglitol (Glyset)
Biguanides	Reduce the amount of glucose your liver makes	Metformin (Glucophage)
DPP-4 inhibitors	Improve your blood sugar without making it drop too low	Linagliptin (Tradjenta), saxagliptin (Onglyza), and sitagliptin (Januvia)
Glucagon-like peptides	Change the way your body produces insulin	Dulaglutide (Trulicity), exenatide (Byetta), and liraglutide (Victoza)
Meglitinides	Stimulate your pancreas to release more insulin	Nateglinide (Starlix) and repaglinide (Prandin)

SGLT2 inhibitors Release more glucose into the urine Canagliflozin (Invokana) and dapagliflozin (Farxiga)

Sulfonylureas Stimulate your pancreas to release more insulin Glyburide (DiaBeta, Glynase), glipizide (Glucotrol), and glimepiride (Amaryl)

Thiazolidinediones Help insulin work better Pioglitazone (Actos) and rosiglitazone (Avandia)

You may need to take more than one of these drugs. Some people with type 2 diabetes also take insulin.

Gestational diabetes

You'll need to monitor your blood sugar level several times a day during pregnancy. If it's high, dietary changes and exercise may or may not be enough to bring it down.

According to the Mayo Clinic, about 10 to 20 percent of women with gestational diabetes will need insulin to lower their blood sugar. Insulin is safe for the growing baby.

Diabetes and diet

Healthy eating is a central part of managing diabetes. In some cases, changing your diet may be enough to control the disease.

Type 1 diabetes

Your blood sugar level rises or falls based on the types of foods you eat. Starchy or sugary foods make blood sugar levels rise rapidly. Protein and fat cause more gradual increases.

Your medical team may recommend that you limit the amount of carbohydrates you eat each day. You'll also need to balance your carb intake with your insulin doses. Work with a dietitian who can help you design a diabetes meal plan. Getting the right balance of protein, fat, and carbs can help you control your blood sugar. Check out this guide to starting a type 1 diabetes diet.

Type 2 diabetes

Eating the right types of foods can both control your blood sugar and help you lose any excess weight.

Carb counting is an important part of eating for type 2 diabetes. A dietitian can help you figure out how many grams of carbohydrates to eat at each meal. In order to keep your blood sugar levels steady, try to eat small meals throughout the day. Emphasize healthy foods such as:

- fruits
- vegetables
- whole grains
- lean protein such as poultry and fish
- healthy fats such as olive oil and nuts
- Certain other foods can undermine efforts to keep your blood sugar in control. Discover the foods you should avoid if you have diabetes.

Gestational diabetes

Eating a well-balanced diet is important for both you and your baby during these nine months. Making the right food choices can also help you avoid diabetes medications. Watch your portion sizes, and limit sugary or salty foods. Although you need some sugar to feed your growing baby, you should avoid eating too much. Consider making an eating plan with the help of a dietitian or nutritionist. They'll ensure that your diet has the right mix of macronutrients. Go here for other do's and don'ts for healthy eating with gestational diabetes.

Diabetes diagnosis

Anyone who has symptoms of diabetes or is at risk for the disease should be tested. Women are routinely tested for gestational diabetes during their second or third trimesters of pregnancy. Doctors use these blood tests to diagnose prediabetes and diabetes:

The fasting plasma glucose (FPG) test measures your blood sugar after you've fasted for 8 hours.

The A1C test provides a snapshot of your blood sugar levels over the previous 3 months.

To diagnose gestational diabetes, your doctor will test your blood sugar levels between the 24th and 28th weeks of your pregnancy.

During the glucose challenge test, your blood sugar is checked an hour after you drink a sugary liquid.

During the 3 hour glucose tolerance test, your blood sugar is checked after you fast overnight and then drink a sugary liquid.

The earlier you get diagnosed with diabetes, the sooner you can start treatment. Find out whether you should get tested, and get more information on tests your doctor might perform.

Diabetes prevention

Type 1 diabetes isn't preventable because it's caused by a problem with the immune system. Some causes of type 2 diabetes, such as your genes or age, aren't under your control either. Yet many other diabetes risk factors are controllable. Most diabetes prevention strategies involve making simple adjustments to your diet and fitness routine. If you've been diagnosed with prediabetes, here are a few things you can do to delay or prevent type 2 diabetes:

Get at least 150 minutes per week of aerobic exercise, such as walking or cycling.

Cut saturated and trans fats, along with refined carbohydrates, out of your diet.

Eat more fruits, vegetables, and whole grains.

Eat smaller portions.

Try to lose 7 percentTrusted Source of your body weight if you're overweight or obese.

These aren't the only ways to prevent diabetes. Discover more strategies that may help you avoid this chronic disease.

Diabetes in pregnancy

Women who've never had diabetes can suddenly develop gestational diabetes in pregnancy. Hormones produced by the placenta can make your body more resistant to the effects of insulin. Some women who had diabetes before they conceived carry it with them into pregnancy. This is called pre-gestational diabetes.

Gestational diabetes should go away after you deliver, but it does significantly increase your risk for getting diabetes later. About half of women with gestational diabetes will develop type 2 diabetes within 5 to 10 years of delivery, according to the International Diabetes Federation (IDF).

Having diabetes during your pregnancy can also lead to complications for your newborn, such as jaundice or breathing problems. If you're diagnosed with pre-gestational or gestational diabetes, you'll need special monitoring to prevent complications. Find out more about the effect of diabetes on pregnancy.

Diabetes in children

Children can get both type 1 and type 2 diabetes. Controlling blood sugar is especially important in young people, because the disease can damage important organs such as the heart and kidneys.

Type 1 diabetes

The autoimmune form of diabetes often starts in childhood. One of the main symptoms is increased urination. Kids with type 1 diabetes may start wetting the bed after they've been toilet trained.

Extreme thirst, fatigue, and hunger are also signs of the condition. It's important that children with type 1 diabetes get treated right away. The disease can cause high blood sugar and dehydration, which can be medical emergencies.

Type 2 diabetes

Type 1 diabetes used to be called "juvenile diabetes" because type 2 was so rare in children. Now that more children are overweight or obese, type 2 diabetes is becoming more common in this age group.

About 40 percent of children with type 2 diabetes don't have symptoms, according to the Mayo Clinic. The disease is often diagnosed during a physical exam.

Untreated type 2 diabetes can cause lifelong complications, including heart disease, kidney disease, and blindness. Healthy eating and exercise can help your child manage their blood sugar and prevent these problems.

Type 2 diabetes is more prevalent than ever in young people. Learn how to spot the signs so you can report them to your child's doctor.

Cbd oil for diabetes

Diabetes is a disease where your blood sugar, also called glucose, is too high. Although according to scientific and anecdotal reports CBD for diabetes is more effective and safer, than pharmaceutical medicines, it is still rather unknown. More than 100 million people in the United States have diabetes or are prediabetic, according to the CDC (Center of Disease Control and Prevention). According to the same report, 30.3 million Americans—nearly 1 in 10—have diabetes.

The World Health Organization predicts that by 2030 the number of people with diabetes will double. If we take a look at the history of diabetes in the last decade, the number of people diagnosed with diabetes jumped by almost 50 percent. This indicates that diabetes is not some kind of "abstract, mysterious" illness.

According to the CDC nearly 16% of adults diagnosed with diabetes were smokers, nearly 90% were overweight and more than 40% were physically inactive.

Diabetes is likely caused by society's external impacts. Since we know that it's a metabolic disease, by default we conclude that the highest risk of being diagnosed as diabetic is due to one's individual lifestyle and nutrition.

From 2011 to 2015, diabetes in canines increased by 32%. Luckily cannabidiol dog oil works just as well for humans as it does for dogs and a significant improvement of the diabetes condition can be achieved.

CBD Impact on Diabetes

Even though the public is more scared of AIDS, we have more people dying from Diabetes than HIV. It's no wonder, when even an average medically-informed person knows that diabetes causes kidney failure, blindness, amputations, heart failure and stroke. Before we jump into the scientific, clinical, and anecdotal studies, let's start with one of CBD's effects and CBD oil benefits. Besides commonly known effects like pain relief with CBD, CBD is known as the natural remedy for diabetes.

"Unlike insulin, CBD diabetes treatment may actually suppress and perhaps cure the disease," – Mark J. Rosenfeld, CEO of ISA Scientific. Are you interested in knowing what the leading CBD oils for pain and anxiety are? Follow the links for comparison studies.

Laboratory Studies

One of the best and most trusted studies is a result of many years of research and testing done by scientists Raphael Mechoulam and Ruth Gallily from the Hebrew University. This research clarified that CBD can treat the inflammation caused by a sugar-imbalance in the blood.

At first, scientists focused on the discovery of how insulin unlocks cells and lets glucose enter so that it can activate the energy that our body needs. Then, they distinguished between Type 1 and Type 2 Diabetes. In addition, experiments on rats treated with CBD show the involvement of the endocannabinoid system.

Cannabinoid receptors have been identified in the pancreas, which automatically means it plays a role in decreasing the severity of diabetes. This is the process in which cannabinoid receptors play an essential role in the pancreas the insulin producer that our body depends on for energy.

Another important and strong piece of evidence from the experiment on rats is that CBD has a positive impact on decreasing inflammation of pancreatic cells. Results from a study conducted on rats with infarcts (areas of dead tissue) due to a blood supply failure showed that after CBD treatment, the infarcts were reduced by 30%.

Diabetes Type 1 and Diabetes Type 2

A study conducted in Israel in 2015, led by Raphael Mechoulam, indicated that the anti-inflammatory properties of cannabidiol could treat both diabetes type 1 and 2. A year later, in 2016, the improved research showed that an experimental CBD treatment reduced inflammation in the microcirculation of the pancreas in mice.

An autoimmune disease study, published in 'Autoimmunity Journal', drafts that injections of 5 mg per day of CBD significantly reduced the level of diabetes in mice. The same team went even further and reported that 60% of the mice treated with CBD remained diabetes-free for 26 weeks, in comparison to those without CBD treatment.

How did CBD succeed in decreasing inflammation in mice? Quite simply, it's the anti-inflammatory properties of cannabidiol. Another study on rodents at the Medical College of Georgia discovered that the CBD cannabinoid protected eyes from retinal cell death and breakdown of the blood-retinal barrier. Lead scientist, Dr. Liou explained, "What we believe cannabidiol, as an antioxidant, does is to neutralize the toxic superoxides. Furthermore, it inhibits the self-destructive system and allows the self-produced endogenous cannabinoids to stay there longer by inhibiting the enzyme that destroys them."

Clinical Studies

First of all, clinical trials confirmed that both CBD and THC are "safe profile" compounds which can effectively treat a metabolic disorder such as diabetes.

Clinical trials also confirmed that CBD plays a major role in decreasing and treating both diabetes type 1 and type 2. When it comes to diabetes type 1, one of the studies in the US also confirmed this. Patients who were treated with cannabis had 16% lower fasting insulin levels, and 17% of insulin resistance. The examined non-users didn't experience the same progress. The rest of the studies in this category also endorsed the fact that CBD is a stronger antioxidant than vitamin E or C.

A UK research team launched a clinical pilot trial to examine the CBD effect in type 2 diabetes patients. The method they used was a placebo-controlled and double-blinded format. The examined group received a dosage of 100 mg twice daily for the duration of 13 weeks. The targets were patients with type 2 diabetes.

The results were great; a change in HDL-cholesterol concentration, insulin sensitivity, body weight, glycemic control, lipid profile and very important markers of inflammation were observed. A British company GW Pharmaceuticals also included CBD in a type 2 diabetes trial. The results showed an improved insulin response and greater pancreatic cell function as well as significantly reduced blood pressure levels.

A study under the name "Marijuana in the Management of Diabetes" confirmed that cannabis users are less likely to become obese. Additionally, another finding is that cannabis or CBD users develop "good cholesterol" and have better carbohydrate metabolism than non-users.

Clinical Trials in the Pipeline

Based in Israel, ISA Scientific has launched a global collaboration and licensing agreement in order to advance CBD therapies. In a statement, ISA Scientific CEO Mark J. Rosenfeld said, "The licensing agreement is very well timed because our Phase 1 clinical trials on dosing and safety are now underway in Israel and arrangements for Phase 2 trials for treating diabetes are in process."

Anecdotal Studies

CBD hemp oil is a life-savior and this has been and is still being confirmed by strong anecdotal evidence. The result that, patients find to be the most impressive is that CBD is the key factor for establishing homeostasis, in other words; stable internal functioning despite fluctuations in the external environment. One of the patient stories is about C.W., a 36 years old man in California diagnosed with type 1 diabetes. He is living proof that Cannabis and CBD helped him with the complications such as "Diabetic Retinopathy". With the advice of a doctor and with an official recommendation for using marijuana, this patient took control of his blood sugar and other diabetic complications.

The treatment confirmed CBD's effect of reducing oxidative stress on the nervous and circulatory systems. Time Magazine reports the endorsement by the Harvard Med School researcher Murray Mittleman that current diabetic patients on CBD treatment witness a gradually normalized blood-sugar level.

CBD Oil Dosage for Diabetes

On this site, we always indicate the dosage amount in milligrams CBD. The number of drops varies per product because of different concentration levels. If you take the number of milligrams as your dosage unity, the concentration basically does not matter. For the same milligram dosage, the number of drops may vary depending on brand and type.

With very high dosage levels and low concentration oils, you will have to take many drops. Therefore, often in these situations, people use higher concentration oils. Besides that, almost always, the higher concentration oils are more priceworthy.

The first thing that a patient should consider when it comes to dosage for CBD diabetes treatment is the severity of the condition. People with mild issues require less dosage than those with more severe conditions.

CBD Dosage for Mild Diabetes Symptoms

For Mild diabetes conditions, people usually take 40 to 50 milligrams CBD daily and monitor their blood-sugar level. Based on that they either increase or, decrease with 10-20 mg steps or, if they are satisfied with the results, maintain the same dosage level.

CBD Dosage for Severe Diabetes Symptoms

For severe diabetes conditions, people usually start with 100 or 150 milligrams CBD daily and monitor their blood-sugar level, just like described above. Based on your blood-sugar level you should be able to start decreasing the insulin amounts. Often, diabetes patients can completely eliminate insulin intake after gradually having decreased their insulin.

As a maintenance dosage, to maintain your health-balance or homeostasis, a dosage of 20 to 25 mg is common. Because it is impossible to overdose CBD, you can safely experiment with the dosage level, monitoring the effects and your blood-sugar level.

General dosage guidelines are as follows:

Start small.

Monitor.

Increase if the improvement dynamics are too weak until you see good improvement dynamics.

Decrease when you see strong improvement dynamics and monitor to keep the same dynamics with less dosage.

Keep the same dosage level if you see good improvement dynamics and decreasing results in weakening of the dynamics.

Glaucoma:

A single CBD dose of 20-40 mg under the tongue. Doses greater than 40 mg may actually increase eye pressure.

There are many methods of CBD use. The most common way is in the form of oil or tincture where CBD should be first held under the tongue, to be absorbed in the mouth for at least one minute, before swallowing. This method of intake is called the sublingual intake.

With sublingual intake, some of the CBD taken will be broken down by the digestive system, but most of it will be absorbed by your body directly, shortening the effect lead time. Other oral methods include capsules, mouth strips, and edibles such as chocolate bars.

Many people also enjoy using CBD oil via vaporizers or inhalers as this is a near instant delivery method that can be quite effective, but not as long lasting as sublingual and oral intake. Others use CBD oil by topical skin absorption via lotions, balms, creams or patches.

The amount of CBD can be indicated in different ways on the packaging of different brands. Often, they indicate the number of milligrams of CBD and the total amount of drops in the bottle. This makes it easy for you to calculate how many drops you need to take your daily dosage. If not, just use our CBD calculator.

Besides CBD, THC oil concentrate dosage could help to boost the effects of CBD even further. With cancer treatment, RSO oil is recommended to be used in a mixture with CBD oil.

Best cbd oil for diabetes

Royal CBD

Pros:

Royal CBD uses American-grown, organic hemp

The company uses full-spectrum CBD to make their oils

The oil is available in three strengths: 250mg, 500mg, and 1000mg

Royal CBD extracts are suspended in premium MCT oil for faster absorption

Each batch of product has been tested in a 3rd-party laboratory for potency and safety

Cons:

Slightly more expensive than the other brands

My Thoughts on Royal CBD:

Royal CBD is a company specializing in manufacturing premium CBD oils — made from organically grown US hemp. Unlike many brands that try to make their name in the industry, this company is pretty simple. They offer CBD in basic formats, such as oils, capsules, and gummies.

Their CBD oil is available in three different potency options to address different dosage needs. This is a full-spectrum extract — it contains pure CBD along with other cannabinoids such as

CBG, CBN, CBDA, CBC, and trace amounts of THC (less than 0.3%).

Each batch of their product is tested in 3rd-party laboratories to make sure there aren't any inconsistencies in the CBD potency and purity levels. The results are available on Royal CBD's website.

2. CBDPure

Pros:

CBDPure products are sourced from organic hemp

Extracted with CO2

Lab-tested for potency and purity

100% Satisfaction Guaranteed program (full refund within 90 days)

Cons:

Narrow product range

The oil has a slightly lower strength than the competition

My Thoughts on CBDPure

CBDPure was founded in 2016 by Colorado natives, with a simple mission — to make high-quality CBD oils made from locally grown hemp. The company offers three different strengths of their CBD oil as well as easy-to-take softgel capsules. While this is a very modest product range, CBDPure has perfected both of these products. These full-spectrum extracts are made with supercritical CO_2 and tested in third-party laboratories for potency and purity.

When it comes to their CBD oil, it's not as potent as the other brands in this ranking, but it does a decent job at alleviating mild symptoms or if you use CBD for the extra boost of your health. If you want something potent, you can go for their softgels — each capsule has 25mg of full-spectrum CBD.

If you're not satisfied with your product, CBDPure has a 100% Satisfaction Guaranteed program. They will give you a full refund if you send your order back within 90 days.

3. Hemp Bombs

Hempbombs 300mg oil bottle

Pros:

This company uses certified organic hemp from European farms

Their CBD isolate is extracted with CO_2

Extremely potent — up to 4000mg of CBD per bottle

Extensive product range

THC-free

Odorless and flavorless

All products are tested in 3rd-party laboratories for potency and purity

Cons:

This is a CBD isolate — you don't get the synergy from other cannabinoids

Most people don't need such high doses of CBD

My Thoughts on Hemp Bombs:

Hemp Bombs is a great choice for people looking for high-quality CBD isolate and those who'd like to try different CBD formats. The company specializes in making isolate-based CBD products.

Their product lineup features traditional CBD options such as oil, capsules, vapes, and edibles, as well as less common products like CBD-infused beard lotion, tattoo ointment, or syrup. Hemp Bombs gives you more affordable CBD extracts at the cost of some efficacy. Since this is 99% pure isolate, their products don't offer the synergy from other cannabinoids. Thus, the effective dosage may be higher than with full-spectrum CBD.

Nevertheless, if you're allergic to other ingredients than CBD in hemp products, or you must take periodical drug tests at work and can't get a false positive for THC, this is the best company to buy isolate from.

4. CBDistillery

CBDistillery 500mg oil bottle

Pros:

CBDistillery uses Colorado-grown hemp to make their extracts

The company's products are available as full-spectrum CBD or isolate

Wide product range

Each batch of product has been tested in a 3rd-party lab for quality

Their CBD oil is very affordable

Cons:

Their hemp isn't organic

No flavored options available

My Thoughts on CBDistillery:

CBDistillery sells a wide range of CBD products, including CBD oil, capsules, and gummies — available as full-spectrum CBD or isolate (ZERO THC).

The company also has a very impressive potency range for their CBD oil, offering from 250–5000mg of CBD per bottle. Their products are good for people looking to buy inexpensive CBD oil without compromising its quality — the 250mg bottle costs only $20.

Although CBDistillery doesn't use organic hemp in their extracts, the plants come from domestic growers and are processed with supercritical CO_2 for maximum purity. On top of that,

CBDistillery tests all its products in a certified laboratory for potency and potency and safety.

5. NuLeaf Naturals

Nuleaf Naturals 240mg oil bottle

Pros:

The company uses organic hemp to make CBD oil

These are full-spectrum extracts — you get the synergy from other cannabinoids

NuLeaf products are tested for potency and safety in a 3rd-party lab

Available in 5 different sizes — you can get yourself supplied for months to come

Up to 4850mg of CBD per bottle

Cons:

NuLeaf sells only CBD oil for humans and pets

No flavored options available

Slightly more expensive than the market's average

My Thoughts on NuLeaf Naturals:

NuLeaf Naturals has been selling whole-plant hemp extracts for over 5 years now. The company was established by entrepreneurs passionate about the benefits of plant-based supplements. The company specializes in making clean, potent extracts for both humans and pets. NuLeaf sources its hemp from Colorado farmers who use organic practices for growing their plants.

NuLeaf Naturals may not offer the widest product range out there, but they make up for it with the multitude of different sizes to choose from. Their high-grade full-spectrum CBD oil is available from 240mg to 4500mg per bottle.

Choosing the largest option will get you supplied for months. However, the potency remains the same regardless of the size offering 2.4 mg of CBD per drop.

Final Thoughts on Finding the Best CBD Oil for Diabetes

Diabetes is a serious disease and so are its complications. If you fail to take control of your blood sugar, you can end up with severe health consequences.

Numerous studies suggest that CBD has the potential to relieve and even lessen the symptoms of diabetes. Not only that, but CBD can also delay the onset of type 1, and prevent the development of type 2 diabetes.

If you're considering taking CBD oil to manage diabetes, speak to your doctor about your plans and be sure to discuss the CBD oil dosage for your symptoms. Remember that CBD may need some time to take effect, so stay patient and monitor the effects.

www.ingramcontent.com/pod-product-compliance
Lightning Source LLC
Chambersburg PA
CBHW070822220526
45466CB00002B/741